MARTIN
and Me.

WITHDRAWN

My Life On Hold

....

Anne Louise Larpnel

ISBN

978-1-4602-3965-0 (Hardcover)
978-1-4602-3966-7 (Paperback)
978-1-4602-3967-4 (eBook)

Produced by:

FriesenPress

Suite 300 – 852 Fort Street
Victoria, BC, Canada V8W 1H8

www.friesenpress.com

Distributed to the trade by The
Ingram Book Company

Table of Contents

One morning, a few months after Martin had passed away, I got out of bed and was at a loss as to what to do with the time I now had. Mornings had always been a busy time of the day for Martin and me. While I sipped my coffee and was semi-tuned in to the news, thoughts kept creeping into my head about what I had been doing for these past many years. I wondered if the experience I had gained in caring for Martin might be of some help to others. I ran the idea past my children later that day and their response was encouraging. "Go for it, Mum, we have all learned something from this experience," they said. So with their support, I sat down and started writing.

To my children, M.T. W.A. and B.G. for all their love and support. M.J. and Dr. T. Friends and neighbours, and to my team at FriesenPress. But especially to my lovely, gentle, gentleman husband Martin.

Until the twelfth of never.

This prayer was given to me by my niece shortly after Martin passed away. I carry it with me in my wallet everywhere I go.

One night a man had a dream. He dreamed he was walking along the beach with the Lord. Across the sky flashed scenes from his life. For each scene, he noticed two sets of footprints: one belonging to him, and the other to the Lord. When the last scene of his life flashed before him, he looked back at the footprints in the sand. He noticed that many times along the path of his life there was only one set of footprints. He also noticed that it happened at the very lowest and saddest times in his life. This really bothered him and he questioned the Lord about it.

"Lord, you said that once I decided to follow you, you'd walk with me all the way. But I have noticed that during the most troublesome times in my life, there is only one set of footprints. I don't understand why when I needed you most you would leave."

The Lord replied, "My precious child, I love you and I would never leave you. During your time of trial and suffering, when you see only one set of footprints, it was then that I carried you."

INTRODUCTION

It affects millions of people all over the world, and the numbers keep increasing all the time.

The Government of Ontario is trying to encourage spouses, family members, and partners to take care of their loved ones in their own homes under the Home Care Program. I am talking about Alzheimer's disease and other types of dementia.

I made the decision to care for my husband just over seventeen years ago when Martin was first diagnosed with Alzheimer's disease. This is a horrible, debilitating illness with no known cure as of yet. So I became his caregiver. He passed away in 2013.

I believe the experience I gained throughout those many years might help others who are wrestling with such an important decision that will affect their whole lifestyle.

That is why I have written my personal story about *Martin and Me*.

- 1 -

OUR STORY

I had never thought much about the lifestyle I had with my husband Martin. When my friends said, "You need to get out more," I just laughed at them. Looking back, I can see what they meant.

My son answered the phone one evening. I had just come home from work, and I was busy preparing dinner. "It's for you, Mum," he called. "Who is it?" I asked. "It's a man, and he asked if he could speak to you." I picked up the phone in the kitchen and asked my son to hang up. "Hello?"

"Oh hello, Anne. It's Martin."

"Martin who?" I said.

"It's Martin Larpnel."

My mind was racing. Why was he calling me, and how did he get my number? I had seen him at work but had never actually spoken to him, other than a *hello* or *good morning*.

"You are probably wondering why I'm calling you."

"Well yes, I am."

"I danced with you a long time ago at one of our company Christmas parties, but I didn't know anything about you so I asked one of the other girls you work beside."

I had completely forgotten about that. I had been persuaded to go to the Christmas party by the girls. "You never come out with us," they had said.

Martin went on to say, "She told me you were a very private person, but that you were on your own and had children."

Again, my thoughts were racing. *Where is this conversation going?* I wondered.

"Was there something specific you wanted?" I asked him. "I'm in the process of preparing dinner and I don't have a lot of time."

It sounded blunt even to my ears, but I really did not have a lot of time. My children usually did their homework or whatever projects they were working on for high school, then it was time for bed for us all.

"Well that's just it, I wondered if you would allow me to take you out for dinner one evening?" I was so taken aback, I pulled one of the kitchen chairs over and sat down.

"Why?" I asked.

"I would like to get to know you. I'm on my own, have been for a while. And well, it's so much nicer to eat with someone."

"This has come totally out of the blue for me," I said.

"Do you think you could call me back after we have had our dinner?"

"Yes, of course. I'm sorry to have called you at a busy time."

I could hardly concentrate on preparing dinner. I had put him off. I needed time to think. I had been asked out many times on dates, and not always by single men, but I always turned the invitations

ANNE LOUISE LARPNEL

down. I was bringing up my children on my own, and had been for nearly ten years. I had a good job, which I also happened to love, and I had my own house, albeit with a mortgage. I had become very independent and content with my life. And I was comfortable in my own skin. Even though money was tight, I managed.

"Who was that, Mum?" I was asked.

"Oh, it's just a guy who happens to work for the same company, and he wants me to go out for dinner with him."

"Is he nice?"

"Well the girls at work think he is."

"You never go out or do anything. Maybe you should go."

"Hey guys, wait a minute. I need to get dinner on the table for us and I need time to think. I asked him to call me back, so let's wait and see if he does."

To be honest, I didn't think he would call back. Outside of work, I knew absolutely nothing about him or his personal life. I didn't listen or take part in office gossip. We had just finished washing up the dinner dishes (in our home, we all pitched in) when the phone rang. It was him.

"Hi, Anne. It's Martin again. I hope I'm not interrupting you? Did you give any thought to what I asked you?"

"Yes, but I have to be honest with you. I don't know anything about you outside of work," I said.

"Well, my children are grown up and have left the nest. I've been living on my own for some time now. I have gone out on a few dates, but nothing to write home about. I enjoy going out for a meal, and it's so much more enjoyable with company."

My children were watching and hanging onto every word. After a pause I told him that if I agreed to go out for dinner, I would meet him, but that I would drive myself. It was summer, and the nights still had a lot of daylight. My insistence on driving myself did not put him off. We agreed on a place and picked a working day. My reasoning was we would both have to work the next day, so I could easily avoid a late night. We said bye and hung up the phone.

The smiling faces that had been listening were quite excited about the whole thing. As for me, all I could think was, *What have I just agreed to do?* I could feel a case of cold feet coming on.

We met in the parking lot of the restaurant where we were going to have dinner. I had chosen an off-white classic line dress and tan shoes with matching purse. I decided on gold earrings and a gold chain for my neck. He looked very smart, I thought. He was about six feet tall. He had on a well-tailored, obviously made to measure, taupe coloured suit (which looked really good on his broad frame) with a cream shirt, a very nice striped tie, and brown shoes.

We ordered our meal, and while we waited for it to arrive we drank our coffee. He told me quite a lot about himself, and I shared a few things about myself, but not everything. I wasn't ready to do that. I ordered chicken and Martin ordered lemon sole. I remember thinking to myself at the time, *We are neither fish nor fowl*. The chicken was delicious, so tender and juicy. Martin remarked it was the best lemon sole he had tasted in a long time. He was a big fish lover.

We seemed to have a lot in common, but it was obvious to me at least, this would be my one and only date with him. I was boring and certainly out of practice. I had not been on a date since my marriage had broken up, and that was nearly ten years ago. I thanked him for a lovely dinner and we parted company in the parking lot.

My nosey children wanted to know how everything had gone. What did we talk about? What did we eat? Was I going out with him again? I told them, adding that I didn't expect he would ask me to go out with him again. I didn't think I was his type. However, it was a few weeks later when he called again, and I found myself

ANNE LOUISE LARPNEL

agreeing to a second date. I think I was probably flattered that I had been asked out on a second date.

We went back to the same restaurant, and this time we were shown to a corner table that was a bit more private. We talked our way through the whole meal, and I found him very interesting. He had very blue eyes and his hair was grey with a side parting. He had a very strong and honest looking face. His voice was deep but soft, and I found it easy to listen to. Once more, we parted company in the parking lot.

The next time I went out with him he asked if he could pick me up at home. "We could have dinner and then take in a show in Stratford, if you like?"

"Okay," I said.

Mikado was playing. I thoroughly enjoyed the night out at the theater, but I did not keep the program so I cannot tell you who was on stage that night. Even though I was growing more comfortable with him, I kept my guard up. There always seemed to be a few weeks between dates, and I wondered about this. I thought perhaps he was seeing someone else at the same time he was seeing me. I decided I would ask him about this. He explained he knew I had been hurt deeply and didn't want to rush me or scare me off. When he dropped me off at home, my children were standing at the front living room window with big silly grins on their faces, watching to see if we would kiss.

We kept our relationship very quiet and private until one time, sitting in our favourite restaurant, we were spotted by one of his colleagues who happened to be there. "Don't worry. I'll have a word in his ear," said Martin. It must have worked, because for the longest time we enjoyed our secret.

We had been seeing each other for a couple of years when Martin began talking about getting married. I backed off. I wasn't ready to give up the life that I had built for my children and me. I had also built a six-foot defence wall around myself. However, to his credit, he didn't give up. He was a quiet, mild-mannered, good-natured, even-tempered man, and I think his stubbornness and persistence won me over. I had talked this over with my children—after all, it would affect their lives, too. It wasn't until the third time he asked me that I said yes. He put his hand in his pocket and brought out a small box. When he opened it, I had to gasp. The ring was beautiful. It was a sapphire surrounded by diamonds. "I have been carrying this around with me, now, for almost a year," he said, grinning from ear to ear.

A few months later we were married. It was a small wedding with my girlfriend as my Maid of Honour and her husband as Martin's Best Man. And the rest, as they say, is history.

Even though we had very different personalities, we complimented each other in many ways. Martin was quiet and thoughtful and always a gentleman. He could sometimes be impulsive, especially when it came to shopping. I, on the other hand, didn't care much for shopping, particularly for clothes. I preferred to make my own and sometimes would sew something for Martin. He enjoyed a good joke and had the heartiest laugh I have ever heard. We enjoyed travelling, golfing, dancing, singing, walking along beaches or hills or through small villages. When the weather was inclement, we were just as comfortable staying indoors and reading a good book. Our days were always full and interesting. It was rare that we ate out, as Martin preferred to eat at home and I enjoyed cooking for him. He never failed to compliment on the meal he had just eaten, and he often asked for seconds.

We had been happily married for nine years when I began to notice a difference in Martin. It was very subtle, in the beginning. Hardly noticeable.

"Where are my car keys?" he would ask.

"Have you seen my wallet?"

I didn't think much about these small incidents. After all, everybody forgets things from time to time. But as time went on, these types of questions became more frequent and varied.

Martin had been a professional man in his working career, and so it was one evening as we were about to attend a dinner for a retiring colleague when he asked me, "Where are we going?" He was annoyed with himself, and wrapping his arms around me he asked, "What is happening to me?"

I kissed him and whispered, "We are just getting older." But I sensed there was more to it than that, and so did Martin. We carried on with our day-to-day living and continued to go on our holidays, but I was paying a lot more attention to his behaviour. He was still forgetting things more and more, but now he was putting the teapot in the fridge or not closing the curtain while he was having a shower—needless to say, there was a flood to mop up. Martin knew that things were not right, and as he became more aware, he grew less talkative and no longer took part in conversation when our friends would visit. I often caught myself watching him and would think to myself, *He is somewhere else inside his mind. How can I reach him to help?*

I made many subtle hints about seeing our family doctor, using the excuse that it was time for his annual physical. But these suggestions fell on deaf ears. He became more and more withdrawn and would get quite frustrated and annoyed with himself when he was unable to do simple, everyday tasks like tying his shoelaces or buttoning up his cardigan. One day, when we were out in the car, I glanced over at him and saw that he had only shaved one side of his face. Another time, he had two different shoes on his feet. This he didn't seem to mind too much. He would laugh and shrug his shoulders. But what did frustrate him—and at times me, too—was when he would ask a question that I would answer, and then a few minutes later he would say, "I know I've asked you this already," and ask the same question again. His attention span was getting shorter, and the many subjects that usually caught his attention didn't seem to grasp his interest anymore. Our conversations became more about the past than the present or the future. We started doing more crosswords, played jeopardy and trivial pursuit. We did jigsaws and any other game I could think of to stimulate our brains. By this time I was sure all was not right with the man I loved and shared my life with, but I was having a tough time convincing Martin to see a doctor. We had always been able to communicate with each other, and Martin had often remarked it was my honesty and integrity that had attracted him to me. Now I felt I was being put to the test. *Should I continue to try and convince him to see a doctor, or should I take the bull by the horns and make an appointment?* I chose the latter.

-2-

THE DIAGNOSIS

One week later, as we sat in the doctor's waiting room, Martin asked, "Why are we here?"

"I thought we were due a visit," I said, and that seemed to satisfy him. When I made the appointment, I had quickly explained some of what was happening and passed a note to the secretary with some of my own thoughts for the doctor, so when Martin's turn arrived, I let him go in to see the doctor alone. It seemed like forever, but of course it wasn't long before the doctor poked his head out and motioned me to join him. He explained he had given Martin a physical exam and everything seemed good, but he believed a scan might clarify some queries that he had regarding Martin's memory lapses. He also encouraged us to carry on as normal, but cautioned me never to leave him on his own. I knew what this meant and agreed with the doctor that with a few adjustments, this would not be too difficult. The doctor advised us that his office would make an appointment and let us know when Martin should go for his scan.

We didn't talk very much in the car on our way home. My stomach was in knots. As soon as we were inside the house, I went straight to the kitchen, put the kettle on, and made a cup of tea for each of us. Martin was first to break the silence. "What is wrong with me?" he asked. He was looking straight at me with his clear blue eyes, and I knew he wanted the truth. I took a sip of my tea. My cup clattered on the saucer as I tried to place the cup down gently. I got out of my chair and walked around to the other side of the table. As I stood behind his chair, I hugged him and kissed his neck and cheek. I pulled a chair over and sat down close to him. As we locked eyes I told him we would have to wait and see what, if anything, the scan revealed. As I carried on I said, "It's possible you could have Alzheimer's disease or some other kind of dementia. Regardless, whatever the outcome, we will handle it together."

Our next appointment with the doctor confirmed my worst fears. The doctor talked us through what the scan showed. Martin didn't seem to have any questions, but I wanted to know what would be our next step, the best way to proceed, and how to move forward. Alzheimer's disease is a progressive and debilitating illness. It is a neurological disease that kills brain cells. There is no cure as of yet.

On our way home, Martin said, "Let's keep this to ourselves for a while." I agreed, but added, "How about on a need to know basis." Martin accepted this as a common sense thing to do, and with that he said, "Bummer." I don't recall him ever really saying anything else on the subject, and I never heard him complain about the hand he had been dealt. That night, after dinner, I broached the subject gently. I spoke frankly with Martin because I knew he would expect nothing less from me. Thoughts had been racing through my head at the dinner table, and I felt it was important to talk about these thoughts that kept popping into my head while we still could. "Martin, would you ever want to go into a nursing home?" His immediate answer was, "No." "Okay, honey, then you will stay at home here with me, and I will take care of you. If I need to get help, I will get it." I never asked this question again, and it was never discussed again—definitely not between Martin and myself. So we settled back into our day-to-day living.

To anyone going into their doctor's office facing this kind of diagnosis, I can only say go in hoping for the best, but be prepared for the worst. Discuss everything that is relevant to your lives—health care,

ANNE LOUISE LARPNEL

special needs, finances, legal issues that might crop up, available help, changes to your lifestyle—and try to plan for what lies ahead. It would be prudent to have these discussions while you still can. Try and read as much material as you can get on this subject. Keep in mind that the initial warning signs may be similar, but everyone is different with this disease, and you will be constantly adjusting to whatever is going on with your loved one.

In our case, as Martin's illness progressed, I would try and explain everything as best I could to him. Whether I was helping him to do something that he was having a problem with or when he could no longer do anything for himself, this was something I continued to do all the way through until the end. Perhaps, this is why he never got aggressive with me.

Always let your loved one know what you are about to do, and explain why before you do it.

- 3 -

DAY PLANNING

Unless we had planned something the night before, when Martin and I got up in the morning, we would talk about what we would do that day while eating our breakfast. Sometimes I would pack a lunch and off we would drive to the beach for a picnic. Another day we would pick a village and spend a good part of the day walking around. Often, if there was a tearoom or cafe, we would go inside and enjoy whatever they had to offer. If there happened to be an antique shop, we would go in and look around. We loved doing this and sometimes come out with some article that had caught Martin's eye. We would plan for a day at the art gallery or museum. Martin loved Shakespeare. I, not so much. But we would compromise. I would go with him to a Shakespearian play, and he would come with me to watch a more modern show. We both loved musicals, so there was no disagreement there. On the way home we'd sing songs from the show we had just been to see. On the days it rained, Martin would read and, if I didn't have a book to read, I would sew. We would do some gardening, though it was usually me that did the planting. Martin would dig the hole for me, and I would drop the shrub or plant into it. We pretty much did everything together. But then again, we enjoyed each other's company. I loved when Martin was reading a book and would say to me, "you would really like this, love." That's when I would sit on the chesterfield and, getting nice and comfy, ask him to read it to me. I loved when we did this.

He had such a lovely, deep but soft, rhythmic and soothing voice. I found it very relaxing, and there was something intimate about it.

When the weather was still nice enough, we'd go for walks or play a game of golf. We were duffers and really looked to the game as exercise. Martin had a wicked slice. I usually ended up in the rough. Sometimes we played eighteen holes, and other times we would play only nine. It depended on whether Martin was having a good day or a bad one. We never played on the weekend, as that was when the serious golfers were out. So we played weekdays.

We kept ourselves busy and tried to make each day as interesting as possible. This was going to be a learning curve for our family and us. We had no idea how fast this disease would progress, and there didn't seem to be anyone who could tell us.

After Martin's diagnosis was confirmed, I knew I would have to make a few tough decisions. The first one was to take away his car keys. He loved driving, and it was obviously a big part of his independence. I usually sat beside him and enjoyed the scenery go by, but now I would have to take over that task. Problem was, how was I going to accomplish this without Martin getting upset or thinking that he was perfectly fine to drive? Telling someone they cannot drive a car or any kind of vehicle anymore, for whatever the reason, is hard to do and it can be very hard for that person to accept.

I picked Martin's keys up from the tray where he usually left them. I kept this to myself. We weren't going anywhere, so I had time to think about how I would approach the subject with him. We still talked at the dinner table, so I decided it was as good a place as any to start. We ate our meal, and over coffee I broached the subject.

"You know since we have found out about your illness, we will have to make a few adjustments."

"Yes"

"Well one of those is that you can't drive the car anymore."

"Are you serious?" He paused. "You got to be kidding me, right?"

"I'll never be as good a driver as you, honey, but it will be safer for you and everyone else out there," I hurried on.

He nodded his head. "Do I have to stop right away?"

"Yes. But just think, now it's your turn to enjoy the scenery and relax, and you can help me with directions when we go out."

He was very quiet, but he seemed to accept that his driving days were over. Later, I thought that was easier than I thought it was going to be. But the next time we were about to go out, it was the first thing he asked as he put his coat on. "Have you seen my car keys?"

I didn't go into an explanation. Rather, I just said, "I thought that I would drive today. It's time I did a bit more behind the wheel."

"Okay."

I thought I had got away with a difficult job, but every once in a while he would ask why he couldn't drive, or why someone else was driving his car. It was at these times I would have to remind him that he could no longer drive because of his illness. "Oh, that's right. What's wrong with me again?"

Again, I would try and explain it to him in a way I thought would not upset him and keep him on an even keel. It usually worked. Once in a while he would rebel, but by keeping my voice calm and taking my time talking him through what was going on, in time he did accept that he could no longer drive.

Going out and leaving your loved one alone at home or outdoors is no longer an option. Your loved one cannot go anywhere without being accompanied by someone. This is very important. It is very easy for someone with this illness to simply go outside and wander away. There is every possibility your loved one will have no idea where he or she is or even know their own name. Your loved one could get on a bus and find themselves hundreds of kilometers away in a very short space of time. The same applies to the home. Being left alone could lead to all kinds of accidents or even disaster, so you will have to apply the same rules. One other thing is to remove any area rugs you may have on your floor. This is a hazard, as it could slip when your loved one steps on it, or your loved one could trip over it.

You have to safe-proof your home as best you can. This is common sense. Our home happened to have an alarm system that beeped a signal when an outside door or garage door was opened. It was a great asset when the grandchildren were young, and it was proving to be a great asset now. This situation can sometimes be frustrating for your loved one and for yourself. It is not always easy. It is at this time when family and friends or even a Patient Support Worker (PSW) can come to the rescue. I used to arrange with a family member to stay with Martin on one of his days off work, so that I could get out for groceries or anything else I had to do. I would schedule appointments in the same way. This is one of the reasons why you need to establish a routine and get yourself organized.

Usually my routine in the morning would start when I got up out of bed. I would make myself a cup of coffee and listen to the news. Then, while Martin was still mobile and still able shower himself, I would get him started, and when he finished I would help him get dried. He had a bad habit of letting the bath towel trail along the floor in front of him, so I was always wary of him possibly tripping over it. Then I would make sure he brushed his teeth and got shaved. I would help him get dressed, letting him do as much for himself as he could, and finally I'd help get his hair combed. While he could still walk, I would walk him to the kitchen table where he would sit and read the newspaper while I got breakfast ready. Martin liked muesli and mixed up his own, adding dried fruits like apricots and raisins. I tried to encourage him to do as much for himself as he was capable of doing and for as long as he could. He always liked to eat healthy foods. What we didn't know at the time was Martin had celiac disease, and his healthy breakfast was doing him more harm

ANNE LOUISE LARPNEL

than good. My cereal was cornflakes, rice krispies, or porridge. Then we would have toast, fruit and yogurt, tea or coffee. This was our usual breakfast, but sometimes on a Saturday or Sunday I would cook a breakfast. Although I didn't usually have coffee first thing in the morning, I loved the smell of brewing coffee in the house. While Martin would continue reading the newspaper, I would make our bed and just tidy up in general. It's strange, but reading the newspaper was one of the things Martin lost interest in very early into his illness.

The remainder of our day was filled with whatever we had decided to do. This was our routine for quite some time, and we hoped that it would continue for a long time to come. But nothing lasts forever, and a few years after he had been diagnosed, he was shuffling his feet and could only walk for a very short distance. This problem was okay inside the house, but it would change how we got around when we went out. However, I felt it was important to get him walking as much as he could. I was still able to get him in and out of the shower, with the help of grab bars and a shower chair to sit on. These items in the shower gave him a sense of being safe and secure. I would walk Martin to his La-Z-Boy chair in the family room and put on the radio for him. While he listened to classical music, I would do the laundry, housework, and any other mundane chores around the house.

- 4 -

MEETING THE SPECIALIST

Our doctor made an appointment for us to see a specialist in the aging process, and so a few weeks later we found ourselves sitting in his waiting room. No one else was there. Martin was taken in to see the doctor, and I was taken into a different room with the nurse practitioner. She was short in height and rather large in girth. I immediately dismissed the thought that had popped into my head as unkind and focused my attention to the matter at hand.

Her first question was, what did I think was wrong with my husband? I replied, "I thought he had Alzheimer's disease." She nodded and proceeded to go down a very long list of probing and personal questions about Martin and me. When she completed her list, I was taken into the same room as Martin and the doctor. Martin looked relaxed, but I could tell he couldn't wait to get out of the office. To be honest, neither could I.

The doctor never used the word Alzheimer's. He referred to Martin as having a tired brain. The appointment lasted two hours. Before we left we were given an appointment to come back in four weeks time and given a prescription for Aricept. We kept these appointments, which became much shorter in time, for a year. I couldn't see what benefit, if any, Martin was getting from them. I made sure he took his Aricept every morning. It was supposed to slow the progression of the disease down, I could only hope and pray that it did.

We had just finished our dinner one evening when the phone rang. "Hello," I said. The voice at the other end of the line sounded young. She introduced herself and explained she was a student at the university and was doing research on people diagnosed with Alzheimer's disease. She wondered if she could speak to Martin and ask him a few questions, it would only take a few minutes of his time. I told her that I was his wife and he was unable to come to the phone, but could she tell me who she was doing the research with. She very kindly gave me the names of two doctors she was working with. I thanked her for calling and replaced the receiver back on the cradle. I repeated the conversation to Martin. Like me, he was very annoyed. Unlike Martin, I simmered on what had just taken place, and as I became more angry I knew I would take it up with the doctor at our next visit, if he was there. The past several visits had been with the nurse practitioner alone. My gut feeling told me he would be there, since I felt sure they would know what had happened on the phone with the university student. We kept our appointment, and I had to hide my disappointment when only the nurse practitioner was present in the room. However, when she was finished asking the usual questions and taking copious notes, the doctor came into the room. They changed seats so that he was now facing us and she was sitting off to the side. He asked a few mundane questions to Martin, which he answered with his usual quiet, steady voice. Then he asked me if there was anything else we would like to ask him. You know how you get the feeling he knows what is about to happen? It was one of those moments. I made eye contact with him, and with a clear voice I said I had a concern that I would like to discuss. He nodded and waited for me to continue, but I hadn't missed the quick exchange of looks between the two of them. I ignored this and quickly got into what I had been stewing inside about since the phone call from the university student. I told him about the phone call and watched while they each feigned surprise and shook their heads from side to side.

My first question: "How did this student know about Martin?"

　　　　　　　　　　　ANNE LOUISE LARPNEL

"Don't know," was the answer from both of them.

"How did the student get access to Martin's medical information?"

"Don't know. Our records are locked up and no one has access to them."

"How did the student get access to our phone number?"

"Don't know," again was their answer.

It was sad and disappointing to watch the two of them. Realizing denial was going to be their plan, I told them I believed access to Martin's medical records had come from their office and with their consent. Lots of head shaking and "No, no, that's not possible," was their reaction. I continued, un-swayed, and said the information had come from no one else, since our phone had an unlisted number. It could have come only from their office. Since I now had their attention, I went on to say that they had given away confidential information about my husband. Our privacy had been invaded, without consent, and had caused considerable emotional stress. I went on to say that I was able to speak up for my husband, but I wondered, how many others had this happened to with no one to speak up for them? When I was finished, the atmosphere in the room was pretty tense, and still they continued to deny and make what I considered nonsense comments. I told them this would be our last visit and to forward Martin's medical records on to our family doctor. My parting shot to the both of them was, "What you did was illegal." The look of horror on their faces was priceless. It was their turn to stew.

We got back out to the parking lot and got inside the car. As I sat behind the wheel, I took a deep breath and started to relax. You can imagine my surprise when Martin leaned over and kissed me on my cheek, then patted my hand as it rested on the steering wheel.

"Feeling better?" he asked.

"Yes," I said.

"Thanks for that. I'm glad I have you in my corner".

I had worried I might upset Martin, but now I felt good. I knew I had done the right thing.

We didn't have call display at that time, so when the phone rang the next day I had no idea who was calling. "Hello—" and before I could say anything the voice answered. "This is Doctor ----------,-," he hurried on as though he might lose his nerve. He admitted that Martin's records and information had indeed come from his office and, without our consent, passed on to the two doctors and the student working on research. He was contrite and apologized several times. He went on to explain he was going on vacation for three weeks—did we plan to do anything about this most unfortunate occurrence? I could feel the hair on the back of my neck rising as I listened. I knew he, along with the others, were now doing damage control. Their insistent denials from the previous day flashed through my head and I could feel the anger in me begin to rise again. When I spoke, I managed to keep my voice calm and quiet, but my stomach was churning. I told him to go on his holiday and to call me when he returned. *Then* I would let him know what action we had decided to take. I put the phone back on the cradle and repeated the conversation to Martin. He smiled. I could only imagine what kind of meeting or phone calls had taken place with his colleagues the previous day. I sincerely hoped they were worried, they deserved to be. We would still have to see our family doctor, but for now, we would try and take up our day-to-day living.

This episode, for me, was all about patient confidentiality, privacy, dignity, and consent. These professionals had broken all of these rules.

Once more we had a doctor's appointment, but this time it was with our family physician. He was a tall, young man—slim built and quiet spoken. We had been lucky to get on his patient list soon after he had opened his practice.

We went into his office together, and after he had examined Martin and given him a small memory test, he turned to me and asked what had happened with the specialist. He said he had received a letter along with Martin's medical records. He handed me the letter to read. I was surprised at his openness when he did this. I had to smile. There was nothing about what had actually happened, and it showed the arrogance of the specialist. Our doctor went on to say, "When you make an error of judgement, or make a disastrous mistake like this one, you fess up immediately. Instead they added insult to injury, and compounded the problem with their denials." He was shocked at what had happened. I asked him if he would take care of Martin. "Of course I will," he said without any hesitation.

He went on to say he thought he was doing the right thing for Martin when he had referred him to the specialist. There was no reason to apologize here, and I said so. We visited our family doctor until I could no longer get Martin in the car. After that point, he came out to visit with us at home.

I feel sharing the experience of what happened early on in Martin's treatment will help other spouses, family members, or partners to be aware of some of the pitfalls in dealing with some people in the medical profession. Some assume they know best and will do anything without consent. Thankfully, they are not all like the ones we encountered.

When someone suffers from Alzheimer's or any other type of dementia, there comes a time when they might not be able to speak up for themselves. That's when they need someone to speak up for them. With this type of illness, they might not be able to tell someone they are being abused or mistreated. That was a big factor for me when I made the decision to keep Martin at home and take care of him.

- 5 -

OBSERVATIONS

Now, if you will let me, I would like to share with you some of my observations over a seventeen-year span of dealing with this life changing disease.

First of all, according to the medical profession, a definite diagnosis can only be confirmed after death and an autopsy has been performed on the brain.

Alzheimer's disease is a neurological and debilitating disease that kills brain cells, thus preventing the body from functioning properly. There are many reasons banded about as to the cause of this disease, but everybody is different with it, and honestly, I don't think those in the medical field know either.

The obvious symptoms, which I believe most recognize, are loss of memory, disorientation, wandering, misplacing articles, depression, aggression, and the loss of cognitive skills when performing simple tasks.

In our case, Martin's condition was slow in progressing, so I had the benefit of planning how I would take care of the man I loved and was married to. When he was first diagnosed, I promised to take care of him in our home. It was important to keep him in familiar surroundings and with familiar and friendly faces.

If I may, let me say to those who want to take care of their loved one. It is a twenty-four hour job, but it can be as easy, or as difficult as, you make it for yourself. It takes a lot of energy, stamina, and a helluva lot of patience and understanding. Taking care of a loved one is not for everybody. It is a learning curve for most people, and things can change on a daily basis. Personally, I didn't think of it as a job. I looked at it as one-on-one care that Martin would not receive if he were in a nursing home. And each day was another day we shared together.

Don't be frightened, that is not my intention. It is not rocket science, just use common sense. Not only is it a life changer for your loved one, but it is a life changer for the caregiver and family.

My own reason for choosing to be a caregiver was simple. I loved my husband, and when he was well and healthy he had treated me like a queen. He had always made me feel special. When we first got married, we joked that whoever was in a wheelchair first would have the other one to push it. So it was down to me. It was now my turn to treat Martin like a king, and to care for and protect his privacy and dignity to the best of my ability.

I read as much as I could find on the internet, and at the mention of Alzheimer's, I was all ears—especially when there was anything on CBC News about a possible breakthrough or the latest update.

As time went on, I observed more changes happening. Our walks got shorter and we played less golf. He had good days and bad days. Once you accept this for what it is, you have climbed a big hurdle. I noticed he did well conversationally when it was one-on-one and when sentences were kept short. It seemed easier for him to follow the conversation. I think when a lot of people are gathered and all talking at the same time, it becomes just noise, and he either had difficulty hearing or was simply overwhelmed. But please, don't stop talking. It's important to keep talking and to keep your loved one engaged with what is going on.

I talked to Martin all the time. When he stopped reading the newspaper, I would read it to him. He would start to read a book and fall asleep. When he awakened, he would go back to the beginning and start again. This went on for some time because he still wanted to do things for himself. He wants to hold on to his independence for as long as he could. Eventually I would read to him, and he seemed happy to let me. I also used audio stories on discs, which I would play for him while I did housework or cooked a meal. I played music every day on the radio for him because he loved listening to the classics and jazz.

He was very quiet and more withdrawn in the company of others. This could sometimes be embarrassing, especially if the company wasn't aware of Martin's condition. Remember, for us it was on a need-to-know basis.

When we would go for groceries, Martin would get quite agitated when we reached the checkout because he thought we were holding up the checkout girl or others waiting behind us. When he would try to do a simple task, but couldn't quite manage, I would try and persuade him to try a different way. This seemed to work. He didn't get frustrated and he didn't get aggressive. Here, I believe the secret is to approach things from a different angle. There is always another way of doing things. Do not keep correcting or raise your voice, just *go with the flow*. It's easier on the nerves, and it saves your energy. Your loved one won't get frustrated or aggressive. Remember: tender, loving care and patience.

Something else I noticed was visitors would talk to Martin in a raised voice as if he was deaf or as if they were talking to a child. A raised voice can cause your loved one to be alarmed. Your loved one may think the person talking is angry and won't understand why.

One visitor actually remarked that Martin's capacity was at the level of a three year old. I was very annoyed and quick to correct this person. I pointed out that Martin was still as intelligent as he had ever been. The difference now was that he could not remember or vocalize in return. It did not mean he could not hear or understand what was being said.

I realized when anyone visited it was a good idea to remind them just to speak in a normal voice, and as one adult to another. A person with any form of dementia is still an adult and should be treated as such. I honestly believe Martin could still comprehend a whole lot more than he was given credit for.

Martin started to put his hands in his pant pockets—this was a new habit for him. He was also tripping, even though there didn't seem to be anything there for him to trip over. He never actually fell, but I started to hold onto his arm or take a firm grip of his hand. This way I had a firm grip on him, just in case he tripped and lost his balance. When he was tired, he would lean to the side just like the Leaning Tower of Pizza. I found that if he sat down for five or ten minutes he could stand up straight again. These anomalies usually happened when he was getting tired, towards the late afternoon.

Meal times took a bit longer. Sometimes Martin managed on his own, and other times he needed some help. Thankfully he still had a very good appetite and enjoyed his food. Bad circulation in his feet and legs was a problem, but raising his feet when he sat down helped considerably. As time went on, walking around stores and waiting at checkouts would cause him to get tired, and his legs would become weak. He would wobble as though he would collapse at any moment. I solved this problem by picking up a wheelchair as soon as we entered a store. Martin would push it until he got tired, then I would get him to sit in the chair and I would push it. This helped us to get out and about until he got a wheelchair of his own. However, it is important to keep your loved one walking as much as possible, otherwise the muscles will atrophy.

Once he had a wheelchair of his own, there was no stopping us. It gave me extra time getting out and about with my loved one. I could drive out to a quiet road in the country and take him for a walk. I didn't have to worry about going to a store and not being able to get

ANNE LOUISE LARPNEL

a wheelchair. We did this for several years, until I could no longer get Martin into the car on my own.

Let me tell you a short story. Martin was admitted to hospital for an unrelated problem. He was a patient for about ten days. No one got him up out of bed to sit on a chair or take him for a walk along the hallway. As a result, he could no longer walk by the time he came home. He had also lost a considerable amount of weight. I was never really sure if the lack of exercise was the reason he lost the ability to walk, or if it was his memory loss—that he couldn't remember how to put one foot in front of the other.

My son and I tried walking him up and down the hallway everyday for weeks, placing one of our feet behind one of Martin's. But we had no success, and it was too stressful on Martin. He never walked again. The other part of this story is that he had been in a different hospital a few years previous. The nurses got him up out of bed every day, and he was walked along the hallway regularly. He could still walk when he came home.

The fact that he could no longer walk created new problems. I could no longer walk him from his chair to the table for meals. I could no longer walk him into the shower every morning. This changed our routine. I now gave Martin a complete bed bath every morning. It took a bit longer than a shower, so I started a bit earlier.

I used the wheelchair more inside our home. Luckily we didn't have carpet on the floors. They were tile and hardwood, so it was easy to push the wheelchair around. He could still do some things for himself, and I encouraged him.

- 6 -

ROUTINE

Since every household is different and marches to a different beat, try and find what works best for you and your loved one, and encourage your family to lend a helping hand. It will ease your workload, and you will have the company of a family member. It is important that you take time to enjoy the company of others.

Usually my routine in the morning would start when I got up out of bed. I would make myself a cup of tea and listen to the news. Then I would get Martin bathed. I was organized, so I gathered everything I needed for this task. It saved a lot of time, instead of going back and forth for some item that was needed.

When bathing Martin in bed, I would start at the bottom half—wash him and put clean disposable underwear on. Then I would change the water and do the top half. This done, I would help him into his wheelchair and wheel him into the bathroom. I would shave him and help him brush his teeth. Sometimes I would notice him looking at his reflection in the mirror. It was as if he was looking at himself and wondering who the man staring back at him was. Then I would comb his hair, and we would have breakfast together. I would offer help if needed. I wanted him to do as much for himself as possible, and for as long as possible.

After breakfast, I would wheel him into the family room and sit him in his La-Z-Boy chair for a short time. It was also a change of view. Remember pressure on the buttocks, so do not let your loved one sit or lay in the same position too long. While Martin sat in his chair, I would then go and change the bed linen and remake his bed. It was important that the bedroom always smelled fresh and clean. I was always conscious of this.

Over time Martin had become incontinent, so it was important—for both of us, really—that he have a bed of his own. It took me a while to get used to the idea that I was no longer sharing a bed with Martin anymore. I purchased an electrical Home Care Medical Bed with remote control. It was a tremendous asset, as it allowed me to adjust the bed to various positions. A new bed also meant rearranging our bedroom. I wanted to be close by at night, in case Martin needed my help. I was afraid that if I was in a different room I might not hear him. I still miss him lying beside me with his arm around me.

The routine was the same for lunch and dinner. Because Martin could no longer walk, I couldn't let him sit for long periods of time. He didn't shift his weight around, so all of the pressure was on his buttocks. To keep him moving, I began something I used to call our "rock and roll time". I would take him to the bedroom and get him into bed. It was really my way of exercising his legs and arms. I was also always checking his body for red spots. He was becoming more fragile, and I didn't want his skin to breakdown and cause bedsores. It's very important to pay lots of attention to the skin, as it can breakdown easily and quickly. They are painful and very hard to heal.

Think of yourself if you have ever had to sit in one position for a very long time—it begins to hurt. And how good does it feels to stand up and move around? The difference is that while you can get up and move around, your loved one might not be able to do this for him or herself. Pay close attention to the skin, and always

ANNE LOUISE LARPNEL

use moisturizer to keep the skin from getting dry and cracked. I will return to this topic a bit later to explain the importance of establishing a routine and the importance of being organized.

Having a sense of humour can be a great way of handling things that could otherwise cause you frustration. I found laughing was a great release of tension, and often a funny moment helped me get through a tough day.

Quite often when I would be giving Martin his bed bath he would pass gas. As I waved my hand about in an effort to get rid of the smell, I would laugh and say, "Thanks for that." This would make him laugh, and the more he laughed, the more he passed gas. Sometimes it was like a machine gun in the room.

You need to be able to laugh when things that happen strike you as being funny, and you need to keep your sense of humour.

Another time I had Martin sitting on the toilet for about fifteen to twenty minutes. Nothing was happening so I said, "Okay, Martin, we will try again another time." I stood him up and walked him over to the bathroom vanity. He held on to the sink to keep his balance while I got him back into his pants. On this occasion, I was standing behind bent over, and in the process of putting his pants back, something hit me on the head. Instantly I gave my head a shake, and there it was—the culprit, sitting on the bathroom floor. I burst out laughing and said, "Why not? Everybody else does."

What is it they say? Timing is everything. He had just had a bowel movement and "crowned me with it." I still laugh when I think about it.

Another time we were sitting in church when Martin passed gas rather loudly, I might say. As we sat there, I tried to ignore it. Luckily for us, a young couple with three children were sitting on the seat in front of us. I watched as the children looked at each other, wondering which one had farted in church and at the same time trying not to giggle. They didn't succeed. Even the parents couldn't help themselves.

My son would often take us for a drive and on one particular occasion he drove us to Stratford. We wheeled Martin around the town, and on our way home we stopped to pick up ice cream cones. Martin loved ice cream. As we carried on our way home, my son looked across at Martin who was sitting in the front passenger seat. He said over his shoulder, "Take a look, Mum," as he nodded in Martin's direction. The ice cream was melting quicker than Martin could eat it. It was all over his face, running off his chin and onto his shirt, then onto his shorts and finally coming to rest on his legs. Of course the odd bump on the road hadn't helped much either. It was priceless, but there would be a sticky mess to clean up and a washing to do.

ANNE LOUISE LARPNEL

- 7 -

ENTERTAINING

Having guests for dinner was great, but it was also a very busy time and a challenge, just like it is in any home. However, now with Martin's illness, I had to do my preparations at various times of the day to fit it into Martin's routine. Very often I would start the night before. It could be preparing vegetables or making dessert. I usually kept it simple with just two guests. It was easier this way, and it gave me time to enjoy the company instead of spending most of my time in the kitchen. When Martin was in his wheelchair and needed help eating, we continued to have close friends for dinner. They understood and did not mind. If they did mind, they would never have gotten an invite.

Christmas time was a much busier time. The Christmas tree was decorated and so was our home. Some of the decorations were older than my children. We would have the family over, so it was a much bigger affair. I would try and get done as much as I could the night before. I would get up out of bed at the crack of dawn on Christmas morning, get the sage stuffing that I had prepared the night before from the refrigerator, and put it in the oven. After I had bathed Martin and we'd had breakfast, I would get Martin comfortable in his bed, as he usually had a sleep at this time of the morning. It would be a long day for the both of us, so it was important for Martin to rest as much as possible. With so many people in our home in one day, even though it was family, it was going to be noisy and busy.

The kitchen would get tidied up, and then I would take a quick shower. Dressed, I would go back into the kitchen and get on with whatever still needed done for our Christmas dinner. By the time this was done, the stuffing was ready to come out and the turkey ready to be put into the oven. The smell of the sage stuffing would waft through the kitchen, to soon be followed by the smell of the turkey. By the time the family arrived the house smelled of Christmas and already they were all hungry with the smell of turkey and stuffing. It was truly a hectic day, but I have to say I loved it and enjoyed the whole day, and was shattered after they had all left to go home. Years later, when Martin could no longer sit with us at the table for Christmas dinner, I would prepare his Christmas plate and give him his meal before any of the others sat down at the table. It was less noisy, now, but still a very enjoyable day. Our children were now scattered in various countries, and so Martin and I had our last Christmas dinner together with only one other family member and three close friends. That said, none of us knew at the time that it would be our last. It was Christmas 2012.

I had been taking care of Martin for about twelve years, doing most of the work on my own. I didn't give much thought to this until Martin started taking an hour, sometimes two, to get through a meal. It seemed that I was spending the whole day trying to get some food and drink into him. Then one day he stopped eating completely. I called our family doctor, and he came to our home to see him. I know it's a rare occurrence these days. Did I say we were lucky to have him?

Anyway, he thought perhaps Martin's time in this world was coming to an end. So did I. We talked about what to watch for, and what to do if it happened. He left me his cell phone number just in case I needed him in a hurry. I still think of our family doctor as one in a million, these days.

I continued my daily routine and tried to coax Martin to eat some food and drink fluids. This predicament went on for just over two weeks, and then one day he opened his mouth and I was ready. The spoon was in his mouth before he could blink. It was a gradual process at first, because I didn't want to overload his stomach after not having anything to eat for a few weeks. So I pushed a lot of fluids, table jelly, and light meals. Gradually he was eating normally again, and always ready for food.

Always have water and juice at the bedside. It's just as important to get fluids into your loved one, as it is food, so he or she doesn't get dehydrated.

- 8 -

GETTING HELP

My children convinced me to get some help in. I can tell you honestly, it took a lot of persuasion to convince me. The Provincial Government of Ontario had started their Home Program to help folks keep their loved ones in their own home. I made a few enquiries and was put in touch with a case manager. She came out to our home, and after some pertinent questions mainly about how much or little Martin was able to do for himself, she agreed I needed some help. She seemed genuinely surprised at what I had been doing on my own. I hadn't given it much thought. I wanted someone to come in at lunchtime and give Martin his lunch. Unfortunately the Patient Support Worker (PSW) would either arrive too late, and I would already have given Martin his lunch, or she just didn't show up at all. One day a male PSW arrived and was pulling on his latex gloves preparing to give Martin a bath. I explained that he was supposed to give Martin his lunch. Somewhere along the line of communication, he had been instructed to give Martin a bath. He settled for giving him his lunch. He was also surprised at Martin's appetite. When your loved one is eating a meal, don't get annoyed if he or she wants dessert first before dinner. What difference does it make, as long as your loved one is eating? With Martin, sometimes he wouldn't eat a spoonful of dinner, so I would offer him a spoonful of dessert, and he would swallow that down, no problem. The next spoonful was dinner. I would tease him about being an old fraud, which usually brought a smile to his face. But hey, he was eating and that was the important thing.

This predicament of the PSW arriving too late or not showing up, with no phone call from the office to let me know, was beginning to frustrate me. Martin was blissfully unaware of the problem. It was important to me that I stick to the routine I had established for Martin's care. It worked in our household, and Martin seemed to benefit from it. I made a call to the case manager and explained what was happening. I cancelled the agency and said I would wait until someone else could be found, possibly with a different agency. Another PSW was indeed found with a different agency, and she worked out fine. She was very patient and considerate with Martin, and she talked to him. She always arrived on time. I think she only missed three days in the five years she came to our home. Two days she was ill, and the third day was due to a bad winter storm—and I got a call from the office letting me know in advance. I suppose it's like everything else. You get good ones and not so good. **But know there is help out there.**

Something else I started doing was, when I was making a stew, I would make enough to do a few meals. I would divide it into containers and put it in the freezer. It's something I used to do when I was still working. This freed up time to do other things. I did the same with casseroles, shepherd's pie, desserts, baking, and puddings. By doing this, I could use the time for something else. Then all I had to do was prepare the vegetables for the evening meal. Our four-legged friend Tramp loved when I did this. He was never allowed people food, but he did enjoy his veggies. Soup was another dish I would make regularly. I always seemed to have a pot of homemade soup on the stove. I would also make wheat and gluten free dishes for Martin. He had celiac disease—his digestive system was unable to utilize fats, starches, and sugar. Studies have shown a deficiency in enzymes that help to metabolize these substances. You would be surprised at the number of products that contain wheat and gluten. But once you know what they are, it's easy to avoid them. These

ANNE LOUISE LARPNEL

wheat and gluten free dishes came in handy if I was having a B.B.Q. I also would stock up on the local berries when they were in season. After washing them thoroughly, I would blend them and then put them into containers, which I froze. I also made popsicles with Jell-O in the summer time, which we both enjoyed. I am sure you did the same thing when your children were small.

I found when Martin was bedridden, and was taking a bit longer to get through his dinner, that I began to have mine earlier rather than waiting until he had eaten his. I didn't like to eat too late, because I felt I was going to bed with a heavy load in my stomach. It is a habit I have had a hard time breaking. I found I was always looking for ways to make my workload easier. In a way, I suppose I had a routine for Martin and one for myself. It allowed me to do things for myself, or to simply put my feet up, while Martin was sleeping. I think I learned to appreciate my spare time more and guarded it jealously.

- 9 -

DEPRESSION

It is my firm belief that anyone with Alzheimer's, or any other kind of dementia, gets frustrated or aggressive because someone is continually correcting or trying to get them to do something he or she does not want to do. Or someone raises their voice or disagrees in an impatient way. Your loved one doesn't know why you are getting impatient. You can correct or raise your voice or show your annoyance till you are blue in the face, but your loved one will have forgotten what all of the raucous was about in minutes. It's much easier on you both to agree more, than to disagree. And smile more than frown. This kind of behaviour can lead to your loved one feeling depressed. Remember: come at things from a different angle. Persuade your loved one to try a different way to accomplish whatever it is he or she is trying to do. A different way to say what he or she is trying to tell you.

Depression is one of those illnesses that can creep up on anyone and take a long time to find out the cause. For someone with dementia it can be as simple as being told that you have dementia. It can also be interpreted as your loved one having a "down day." He or she may be deemed lethargic by the caregiver. It is important for the caregiver to recognize this and to stay positive. You need to be aware and do things that your loved one enjoys doing. Try to keep life interesting and stimulating. It could be that your loved one is tired and needs to rest. As time goes on, you will find that your loved one sleeps a lot more. Sometimes sleep can be as good as any medicine.

Remember: tasks that are easy for you to do may not be so easy for your loved one anymore. You need to make allowances and show patience and understanding. If he or she complains of being fed up, it is important for you to take the time to try and find out why, and if possible, take steps to correct the problem. Look on it as a heads up that your loved one could be depressed. If you have ever been depressed, then you will know it is not always easy to explain why you feel the way you do. Think how it must be for someone with dementia.

Ask your loved one what he or she would like to do on any given day. This small act will give your loved one confidence and the feeling that he or she has a voice and still make a choice. That his or her opinion and input in day-to-day living still matters and has value. It will give a boost to their morale and self-esteem.

Stay cheerful and show that you are interested in how your loved one is feeling. Be patient, and listen to what your loved is trying to tell you, understanding that these issues can take time. It is also possible that because your loved one has dementia, he or she will not remember why they felt depressed. Your loved one is probably having a tougher time than you are trying to cope with what is happening in his or her life.

-10-

HAZARDS

Take a good look around your home, inside and out. You have to take special care for your own safety, as well as your loved one's safety.

Because your loved one may be experiencing difficulty with balance, never let your loved one go up or down stairs alone. Navigating stairs can pose a problem of their own and not just for your loved one. The stairs inside your home should always have a handrail. Make sure it is fastened tightly and securely. Find the best way for you to give your loved one the support needed to get up or down the stairs both inside and outside your home. If you do not live in a one level house or apartment, see if you have an area that could be converted into a bedroom and bathroom causing the least stress and upheaval. We were lucky in that we lived on one level, so the problem of stairs never presented itself.

There are also chair lifts that can be suited to your stairway that may be a great bonus for your loved one, but you need to give these suggestions serious thought before having anything installed. It would never have worked for Martin, because as time went on, I could no longer get Martin into his wheelchair or car without help. I know these are hurdles that have to be addressed, so it makes sense to try and talk to your loved one while you still can. It will also allow your loved one to feel included in the care plan.

Be aware of your financial circumstances. Many decisions made will depend on this when it comes to making changes around your home, if this is the route you choose. These changes could be expensive. Ask yourself: are they really necessary, or is there another way of getting around the problem? On the other hand, none of these changes may be necessary for you. Use your common sense. Enquire if there is any help the government can provide, and avail yourself of all the details required.

Another hazard is machinery and tools. If your loved one is a handyman or handywoman, you will have to keep him or her away from high powered machinery, electrical tools, and any other tools or equipment that could be considered a danger, such as garden tools. However, be tactful and considerate. Remember that every time you prevent your loved one from doing something, you are taking away another piece of his or her independence. Tread carefully.

Martin was not a handyman. Oh, he could hammer a nail into the wall to hang a picture, but for anything else? Definitely not. For me, having to keep tools or equipment out of his way did not pose a problem.

There are many hazards in the kitchen that most of us do not give second thought to, particularly around the stove. Take a good look around and try and make it as safe as you possibly can, in the same way you would if there were young children in your home. Keep knives and scissors and any other sharp utensils out of sight. You will have to make a judgement call as to whether or not your loved one is still capable of making a cup of coffee without scalding his or herself, or if he or she should be anywhere near a stove.

Do not take all of your loved one's independence away in one fell swoop. The last thing you want to do is make him or her feel useless. Patience and understanding can go a very long way. Communicate all the time, and get to know what your loved one can or cannot do. Always offer to help and be there just in case. Keep the situation free of stress, and stay calm.

Your bathroom is another place to keep a close eye on. If you have a bathroom mat, remove it. It is good practice to keep the bathroom door open, even if your loved one is still able to take a bath or shower alone. Accidents can happen, or if you think your loved one is capable of causing his or herself harm, you want to have quick access if the need arises. Keep electrical devices—hairdryers, radios, televisions, anything that can be plugged into an electrical outlet and possibly fall into the bathtub—out of the bathroom. If you keep medication in the bathroom (many people do), it should all be kept under lock and key.

You will be surprised at what you are already doing around your home. Now you are simply reinforcing the things you already do automatically. Now you are more aware of hazards that could cause accidents.

- 11 -

MEAL TIME

Eating or drinking can bring problems of their own. If you have ever had a crumb stuck in your throat, or taken a drink and had it go "down the wrong way," you will know what I am talking about. Coughing and choking can be stressful and can cause panic for your loved one and the caregiver. Give your loved one time to eat, chew and swallow. Do not put large amounts on the fork or spoon at any one time. Use a blender or processor, if necessary. It will help the food to slide down his or her throat easier.

This is a good time to have conversation. It doesn't matter what the topic is about, just keep talking and make eye contact. Even when your loved one is no longer able to talk, he or she can still hear you.

You may find that a straw is easier for your loved one to drink with. Do not rush this task. It takes patience. It doesn't matter if your loved one eats dessert first, then eats dinner. The important point is they are eating. We all have food preferences, our likes and dislikes, so suffice to say a good balanced diet is healthy for everybody. Don't forget to practice good oral hygiene, and remove any dentures when necessary.

Before giving Martin his evening meal, I used to wash and change his underwear. I would straighten out any wrinkles in the sheets— these can cause pressure and lead to skin breakdown. Pressure areas are usually boney areas such as shoulders, elbows, hips, buttocks, knees, ankle bones, and heels. Also, skin rubbing against skin can cause the skin to breakdown. It made sense for me to do this first before letting him eat. That way he wasn't being rumbled around after eating. Then before going to bed myself, I would check to see if he needed changed. Just think: if it were you in that bed, would you like to go through the night feeling uncomfortable or wet? After all, what is the first thing you do for yourself when you get up in the morning, and the last thing at night? You go to the bathroom. Remember to change sheets if necessary.

Do not let your loved one sit too long in one position. Prevention is easier than a cure for decubitus ulcers, known as a pressure sores or bedsores to most people. If confined to a bed, change your loved one's position regularly. Perspiration and incontinence of urine or feces can cause bedsores. Do not let your loved one wait too long before washing and changing underwear. Bedsores are very painful and very difficult to heal.

I actually fashioned a pair of booties without toes from a piece of foam covered with a soft material, which I could fit on Martin's feet to protect his heels and ankle bones. I could even wash them in the washing machine. I could never claim they looked fashionable, but they worked. You can also use pillows as a prop for other areas that may be starting to breakdown (red areas). Make sure you dry in skin folds—skin rubbing off skin can breakdown. Be vigilant.

Get yourself organized. Establish a routine that works best for your loved one and yourself. Do not change this routine, even when you have other company. Simply explain how important it is for your loved one to follow the routine. Don't be interrupted when the telephone rings if you are busy doing something for your loved one. He or she could lose the plot and wonder what it is you are trying to accomplish. It is a good idea to let friends and family know when not to call.

-12-

AFTER THE DIAGNOSIS
HAS BEEN MADE

It is very important to have a one on one, frank and honest conversation with your loved one before inviting family members to participate. Be very sensitive and aware of his or her feelings. Try and establish the way to move forward with your lives, and what will work best for you both. It will not be an easy conversation to have, but a necessary one. Be positive, sensitive, listen and be patient and understanding. Talk about what you both understand about this illness. Ask your loved one where he or she would want to be cared for? As an example, would your loved one want to be cared for at Home or in a Nursing Home as the Dementia progresses? Your loved one's input is very important and has value. You should have this conversation as soon as possible and while an informed decision can be made. When you both have a good understanding of what your loved one wants, then it is time to include family members. Your loved one should also be included in this conversation with the family members. After all if it was you, would you not want to have your say about your care and needs? If this is done while your loved one can take part, it will be much easier as time goes on. There will be fewer arguments with family members and less frustration for all concerned especially your loved one. You do not want to be having disagreements at a later stage. Construct a care plan and be prepared to put that plan into action. Always include your loved one, sometimes family members can forget their loved one is sitting in the same room. This can cause your loved one to feel excluded. And that what he or she thinks, or has an opinion on doesn't matter. Do not all talk at the same time it's confusing and a lot of noise. Have a pen and paper at the ready, then as each family member puts a suggestion forward it can be noted. You do not have to adopt all the suggestions put forward. Filter out the one's that do not apply to your situation or circumstances. Remember this is a new experience and a learning curve for all concerned. Your loved one is an adult and an individual, his or her symptoms and behaviour may be different from others with Dementia. You will have to make allowances and changes accordingly. You may need more family meetings as time goes on. There will be challenges ahead so always keep communication lines open, and always include your loved one, even when everyone thinks your loved one is no longer cognizant of what is going on. It will be a lot easier to make the right decisions. This is about achieving the best care possible for your loved one. Dementia is a life changing illness and it will affect you and your family. But most importantly it will affect your loved one. That is why, it is important to have the conversation as soon as possible. Try to answer as many questions as honestly and openly as they present themselves. You won't have all the answers, but discussing everything will help you reach the right decision for your loved one and you. Here are a few questions you can use to get you started.

Does your loved one want to be cared for at Home or in a Nursing Home?

Are you aware of the preferred Care your loved one wants?

Is there a Community Care Access Centre? (CCAC) HELP.

Are you capable of being the Principal Caregiver?

Are you prepared physically, mentally and emotionally?

Are you aware of your financial circumstances?

ANNE LOUISE LARPNEL

Are you financially able to purchase equipment that may be necessary at a later time? (Financial help from the Government may be available)

What are the benefits of Care At Home?

What are the benefits of a Nursing Home?

Are family members prepared to offer their time and help?

The Decision

Should you decide you want to take care of your loved at home, remember:

- Protect your loved one's privacy, dignity, confidentiality.
- Quality of life.
- Human rights.
- Be honest.
- Always make eye contact.
- Keep talking.
- Use common Sense.
- Patience.
- Understanding.
- Humour.
- Treat your loved one with respect and dignity.
- Ask yourself: how would I want to be treated if it was me?
- Remember, it could be you lying in that bed.
- Stay positive.

These are items you might find you need, if you do not already have them.

- Grab bars in the shower or bathtub
- Shower seat/bath seat
- Non-slip mat for shower or bath
- Reasonably deep basin for giving bed baths

- Soap and deodorant
- Bath towels, and face cloths, or a sponge
- Medical home-care bed with bed rails (electrical with remote control)
- Wheelchair (Remember you may be eligible for financial assistance from Government)
- A hoist (a mechanical lifting device)
- Commode (a regular toilet may be too low, and a commode can also be moved around)
- Disposable underwear
- Mattress protection sheet *
- Latex gloves
- Closed house slippers that won't come off easily (which could cause tripping)
- Bed shirts, instead of pyjamas (I used T-Shirts, which I cut up the middle of the back—it's easier to get on and off)

You may not need some of these items right away, but if you do shop around, you may be able to purchase second hand.

*I cut a piece of heavy duty plastic (the kind builders use) to protect Martin's bed. I had discovered (the hard way, you might say) bought protection sheets didn't quite do the job. I also cut a piece for the front passenger seat of the car. My reasoning was it is easier to clean the plastic than the car seat. Plastic also prevented the build-up of odours, such as the smell of urine, in our bedroom and the car.

I had a hydraulic lift with a sling that was battery operated, and could be recharged. The lift came with two batteries, so when one needed to be charged, I could still use the lift. When I wanted to wash Martin's hair, I would position the sling under him, by rolling him on his side, and then hook it onto the lift and wheel him into the bathroom. Then I would position his head over the sink and wash his hair, after drying his hair I would then get him back into his bed.

Personal grooming is very important for your loved one. It's good for self-esteem and morale. Besides, everyone likes to look their best.

Keep hair clean. I used to give Martin a haircut and then tease him that I had just taken ten years off his age. It would be prudent and sensible to speak to your family doctor about keeping ears free of earwax. You doctor may do this task for you. The last thing you want to do is damage the ear canal. Keeping the ears free of wax will help your loved one to hear better, but be very careful if you do this task yourself. Cut the hair around the ears and nose, if necessary. Cut fingernails—if your loved one scratches and breaks the skin, it can become infected. Cut toenails as necessary. This is easier done if you soak the feet first. You may want to have a Chiropodist to do this for you.

When I was giving Martin a bed bath, once I had the front of his body washed I would place one leg over the other, then lift his arm over his body in the same way as his leg. Doing this allowed me to roll him onto his side without any difficulty.

I used the same method to roll the sling under Martin and lift him up off the bed, so that I could change the sheets as necessary and make his bed. The lift was a terrific asset to have. It was extremely stable and surprisingly easy to manoeuver. The home care medical bed I had was electrically operated with a remote control. I could change Martin's position with the press of a button. It also came with a lever. So if there was a power cut, I could still change the bed position.

The wheelchair was light in weight, but it had to be pushed. However, it was still easy to push and fold up when we would go out in the car. I had decided on this type because Martin could not operate the wheels with his hands or work the electrical type on his own.

Last, but not least.

It is common sense to have a will. If you do not have one, it would be prudent to have one drawn up while you and your loved one can, as soon as possible. Also, speak to your lawyer about Power of Attorney (POA) for Personal Care and Estate. I would suggest that you do not pass this (POA) on to anyone else, providing you are capable and comfortable doing it yourself. It is a great and important responsibility, but it will save you a lot of stress and frustration when the time comes, not just at death, but when your loved one can no longer make decisions for him or herself. This is a very important document to have. If you have to make decisions regarding your loved one's medical care, finances, income tax, etc., it gives you the power to act and speak on his or her behalf. Even If you do not own property, there may be special items your loved one wants a particular individual to have.

-13-

THE DAY-TO-DAY

Bathing Time

Remove all of your own rings or bracelets that could scratch and possibly break the skin of your loved one. Wash your hands with soap and warm water before starting and when finished. Do not leave your loved one alone during this task.

Gather together everything you will need to assist your loved one into the shower or bathtub. Have all the necessary items at close range so that you can reach them easily. Make sure you have a non-slip mat in the shower or bathtub. Grab bars in the shower or bathtub will give your loved a sense of safety, and offer something to hold on to. Also, a chair in either of these places will allow your loved one to sit if they have a balance problem or get tired, and while you are towelling him or her dry. Help with oral hygiene and shaving, if necessary. Do not forget to moisturize skin.

You can have a Patient Support Worker (PSW) come to your home and help you with the task of bathing. It may not be in the morning, but this is something that you can come to an agreement about regarding time of day. Do not forget to ask your loved one regularly if he or she needs to use the toilet. If your loved one uses disposable underwear, check it often to see if it needs to be changed.

Bed Baths

Wash your hands with warm water and soap before starting and when finished. You will need a reasonably deep basin, two face cloths, soap, and towels, a bed protection sheet, disposable underwear, and latex gloves. Vaseline or antiseptic cream will protect buttocks and act as a protective barrier. You can use a bedside trolley to hold these items. Remove top sheet and blanket. This is when you decide which side of the bed to work from. Whatever side you choose, make sure the guardrails are up on the opposite side of the bed. This will ensure your loved one cannot fall off the bed when you roll him or her over. Use one face cloth for bathing the top half of the body and towel dry, then change the water and use the second face cloth for the bottom half of the body and towel dry. This is the perfect time to check the condition of your loved one's skin, look for red spots. If you notice a red area, this could be from pressure. You can use a pillow to take the pressure off. You can attend to this area when you have finished bathing. Don't forget to change positions and check regularly. You will find a method that works best for you whether you start at the top or the lower part. Don't forget the legs and feet. Dispose of water and anything else no longer needed. Put any soiled underwear or protection pads into a plastic bag and dispose of them. Dress your loved one, and if he or she is still able to get out of bed and into a chair, now would be a good time. Help with oral hygiene or shaving. You may need to put fresh linen and bed protection pads on the bed at this time, or you may prefer to wait until after breakfast. Whatever you choose, it is obviously easier to freshen the bed when it is empty.

Lunch Time

Wash your hands and your loved one's hands. This meal can be less busy, but you still need to prepare everything needed before offering lunch. Doing this will give you time to sit with your loved one and talk or help if he or she needs assistance. If you're prepared, you won't be bobbing up and down because you forgot to bring something to the table. When finished, don't forget to wash your hands. Clean up your loved one, if need be.

Dinner Time

You may want to wash and change underwear before starting. Wash your hands and your loved one's hands. Again, make sure you have everything ready before serving dinner. Wash his or her face and hands, and don't forget to wash your own hands when finished. Do not forget to offer fluids to drink with meals and throughout the day, and always have water and juice beside the bed.

Your loved one's hands may not be as steady as they once were. Spills will happen when getting food from plate to mouth. Spills can be cleaned up, so do not show annoyance or get frustrated. Give your loved one the time he or she needs to get through each meal. Be patient and understanding, and save your energy for something else.

Bed Time

When getting your loved one settled for the night, check and change disposable underwear and bed protection pad if necessary. Offer fluids. Straighten out wrinkles and make comfortable for the night.

It is very important that you wash your hands thoroughly when handling food and before or after carrying out a task for your loved one. It could prevent infection. Your loved one is frail and more susceptible and vulnerable at this stage in their life. Also ask visitors or friends who are ill with a cold or flu to stay away.

Remember: there is help out there.

I found as each year went past, it got easier to care of Martin. That may sound a strange thing to say, but I no longer had to worry about him possibly wandering away, or tripping and falling over, or causing a serious accident. I would have much rather had my old Martin back with me, but that Martin was gone. I considered myself lucky that he had no other major health problems. The most was medication once a day for acid reflux. I used to think to myself how ironic life could be. One of the things I admired so much about Martin was his brain, and that was the part of his body that was affected.

I had often heard others talk about other people with dementia, that their face was a mask, they showed no emotion. Not so with Martin. He still made eye contact with me, and I could ask him for a kiss and get one. I could still get a smile. Martin was in a nice zone at the end. He still looked a lot younger than he was, and he didn't have a wrinkle on his face. As for my wrinkles, I had enough for both of us. I honestly believe he could still comprehend a lot and still hear, more than he was given credit for. He just wasn't able to verbalize back. He certainly recognized my voice. Don't ask, "Do you know who I am?" Always tell your loved one who you are. I told Martin first thing in the morning and regularly throughout the day.

I had been caring for Martin for over seventeen years when he passed away, peacefully and without pain in 2013. I couldn't ask for anything more. We had been married for just over twenty-six years.

I don't think Martin would have lived as long as he did had he been in a nursing home, for the obvious reason. He would never have received the one-on-one care. I do not say this to get a pat on the back or show disrespect to nursing homes, I am just stating a fact. I was organized. I had a routine and stuck to it religiously. I truly believe this played a big part in keeping Martin with me that much longer than he might have stayed otherwise.

When I sat down to put words on paper, I had to think about all of the things I used to do for Martin. It was strange at first, because I had established a routine and got myself organized, I did these things automatically.

Did I get tired? You bet. Especially if I had been up during the night. Did I ever think of giving up? Never. Like Martin, I had a stubborn streak in me, too. Would I do it all over again? Yes. Absolutely. In a heartbeat.

It is definitely not mission impossible.

What now? When Martin came into my life, I was truly blessed. When he passed away, my routine went out the window. For weeks after, I would look at the clock and think, *It's time to get him ready for dinner,* or whatever. It was strange being able to just get in the car and go, without having to arrange to have someone stay with him. Still is. Not having him in our bedroom anymore. Not seeing him last thing at night and first thing in the morning.

I have had to make a big adjustment, but I'm getting there. When I visit his grave, I talk to him and bring him up to date with what's going on in the world. Writing my story has been good for me. I have shed a tear and I have laughed. It has kept me busy. But life goes on, so I will take up my sewing hobby again, and I will revisit an unfinished novel I started to write three to four years ago. I hope to take a holiday and visit my grandchildren. I have my lovely memories of Martin, and I will talk to him and ask his advice when I am not sure about something. Without getting maudlin, because he wouldn't like me to mope, I will talk about him with family and friends. With no regrets or complaints, I put my life on hold for many years, so whatever the future may bring, this is my time.

My advice to a caregiver is this: You will get lots of advice from family and friends. Whether you take it or not is up to you. At the end of the day, if you are going to be the principal caregiver, the decision will be yours. Do not be hard on yourself. You do not have to do this alone. Accept help when offered. It will make your life a whole lot easier and give you some time to yourself. Involve your family. I know, sometimes easier said than done. They are probably still in the work force, but unlike you, they are hardly likely to be working twenty-four hours a day, seven days a week. Perhaps they can stay with your loved one and give you a break for a few hours. If they can oblige, use your time wisely. Get your hair done, go shopping, have lunch with a friend, whatever, just do something that you enjoy. You will feel relaxed and you will have recharged your batteries.

During a visit from our family doctor, he once said to me: "I wish I knew your secret." I don't have one. But perhaps my own experience and tips will help someone who may be considering taking on the job of being the principal caregiver for a loved one at home.

My work in caring for Martin is finished. It ended when he passed away in 2013. But you should know there are thousands caring for a loved one at home, just as I did. You never hear about them. They do not get medals or honoured by the Prime Minister, they just go about their daily routine and get on with it. Your accolades and recognition will come from a much higher source.

*   *   *

It is my most sincere hope that if you have read my story, it will give you a better understanding of what you have chosen to do for your loved one. For you, I wish good health and the courage and the strength to face the challenges ahead.

CPSIA information can be obtained at www.ICGtesting.com
Printed in the USA
LVOW13s1008220814

400317LV00001B/7/P